Contents

Introduction

The system of herbal medicine that developed in China differs in several significant ways from European herbal medicine. The most obvious difference is that the Western herbal tradition focuses on "simples," or herbs taken by themselves. In contrast, traditional Chinese herbal medicine (TCHM) makes almost exclusive use of herbal combinations. More importantly, these formulas are not designed to treat symptoms of a specific illness; rather, they are tailored specifically to the individual according to the complex principles of traditional Chinese medicine. For this reason, TCHM is potentially a deeply holistic healing approach. On the other hand, it is both more difficult to use and to study than its Western counterpart.

TCHM is widely used in Asian countries, both in its traditional holistic form and in a simplified disease-oriented version. There have been a few properly designed scientific trials of TCHM, but the evidence base remains highly inadequate. In addition to questions regarding effectiveness, there remain serious safety concerns to be resolved.

Chinese herbal medicine has a long historical tradition, although it is not quite as ancient as popularly believed. Ancient herbology in China focused on potions whose function was part medicinal and part magical, and it lacked a substantial theoretical base. Sometime between the second century B.C.E. and the second century A.D., the theoretical foundations of traditional Chinese medicine were laid, but the focus was more on acupuncture than on herbs. 1 Only by about the 12th century A.D. were the deeper principles of Chinese medicine fully applied to herbal treatment, forming a method that can be called TCHM. This was further refined and elaborated during various periods of active theorizing in the 14th through the 19th centuries. Western disease concepts entered the picture in the 20th century, leading to further changes.

In China today, TCHM is used alongside conventional pharmaceutical treatment. Considerable attempts have been made to subject TCHM to scientific evaluation;

however, most of the published Chinese studies on the subject fall far short of current scientific standards. (For example, they generally lack a placebo group.)

In neighboring Japan, a variation of the TCHM system known as Kampo has become popular, and the Japanese Health Ministry has approved many Kampo remedies for medical use. The scientific basis for these remedies remains incomplete, but several studies of minimally acceptable quality have been reported.

The herb materials used in all these preparations are gathered from wild supplies or cultivated, usually in China (some come from India, the Mid-East, or elsewhere). There are an estimated 6,000 species in use, including nearly 1,000 materials derived from animal sources and over 100 minerals, all of them categorized under the general heading "herbs." Herbs are processed in various ways, such as cleaning, soaking, slicing, and drying, according to the methods that have been reported to be most useful. These materials are then combined in a formulation; the ingredients and amounts of each item depend on the nature of the condition to be treated.

In some cases, a practitioner of Chinese medicine will design a specific formulation for an individual patient, which might be changed frequently over a course of treatment. In other cases, one or more formulas already prepared for ingestion without modification are selected for use. The outcome is monitored, and the determination of whether to continue the current formula, change to another, or discontinue use is made on the basis of actual versus desired outcomes and the obvious or subtle effects of using the herbs.

As a general rule, acute ailments (those that arise suddenly and are to be treated right away) are treated for a period of 1-30 days. If an outbreak of influenza or eruption of herpes virus is caught early enough, a one or two day treatment will prevent further development of the disease. In the case of acute active hepatitis causing jaundice, a treatment of 15-30 days may be necessary. For chronic diseases (those that have persisted for several months or years), the treatment time is often dependent on the dosage used and the ability of the individual to undertake all necessary steps to overcome the disease (perhaps changing diet, lowering stress, and increasing exercise). When a high-dosage therapy is applied, most chronic ailments can come under control (and some are cured) by a treatment of about three months duration. If the daily dosage is lowered (because of inability to take the higher doses), the treatment time increases-perhaps to 6-12 months. Examples of chronic ailments are autoimmune disorders and degenerative diseases associated with aging. In some cases, herbs are taken daily, for an indefinite period, just as some drugs are taken daily. This is typically the situation when there are genetic disorders or permanent damage that cannot be entirely reversed, problems of aging, and ailments that have been left for too long without effective treatment.

The main reason that more Westerners are turning to Chinese herbs rather than local herbs is because of the vast scope of experience in using the Chinese materials. In every province of China, there are large schools of traditional Chinese medicine, research institutes, and teaching hospitals, where thousands of practitioners each year gain training in the use of herbs. The written heritage of Chinese medicine is quite rich. Ancient books are retained, with increasing numbers of commentaries. New books are written by practitioners who have had several decades of personal experience or by compilers who scan the vast diverse modern literature and arrange the results of clinical trials into neat categories.

American practitioners are usually trained at any one of about 45 colleges in the U.S., with a three- or four-year series of courses that include basic Oriental medical theory, acupuncture, and herb prescribing. Certification is offered at the national level and licensing or registration is offered now by most states. Many doctors from China have come to the U.S. and currently offer professional services throughout the country, but most often in the larger cities. Continuing education is provided through numerous symposia offered by the colleges and professional organizations devoted to Oriental medicine. Often, these meetings focus on the treatment of specific diseases or training in the use of a specialized acupuncture technique or valuable herb formula.

Chinese herbs are provided in the U.S. as food supplements, not as drugs. Thus, they are not strictly regulated by the FDA except for monitoring the cleanliness of manufacturing facilities (for those materials made in the U.S.; for the imported items, FDA monitors only the listing of ingredients to help ensure no toxic herbs are being used). Random testing of crude herb materials and herb products made in the U.S. indicate that they are free of harmful bacteria and chemical contaminants. Imported products must be used with some caution, as some of them are problematic, yet get past the investigators. There are a few patent remedies that are labeled with only herb ingredients, but also contain several Western drugs. Some patents from China contain only Western drugs (and say so on the box, in Chinese), but purchasers may be unaware of this because they are told only that this is an effective remedy that came from China. Thus, imported Chinese herb products should be taken solely on the basis of a prescription from a trained health professional.

Chinese Herbal Medicine

Principles of Traditional Chinese Herbal Medicine

Even a basic introduction to the principles of TCHM exceeds the scope of this article. Consider the following nothing more than a taste of this vast medical system.

According to the principles of all Chinese medicine, health exists when the body is balanced and its energy is freely flowing. The term "energy" refers to Qi, the life energy that is said to animate the body. The term "balance" refers to the relative factors of yin and yang, the classic Taoist opposing forces of the universe. Yin and yang find their expression in various subsidiary antagonists such as cold vs. heat, dampness vs. dryness, descending vs. ascending, at rest vs. active, and full vs. empty.

In an ideal state, yin and yang in all their forms are perfectly balanced in every part of the body. However, external or internal factors can upset this balance, leading to disease. Chinese medical diagnosis and treatment involves identifying the factors that are out of balance and attempting to bring them back into harmony. Diagnosis is carried out by means of "listening" to the pulse (in other words, taking the pulse with extraordinary care and sensitivity), observing and palpating various parts of the body, and asking a long series of questions.

It is important to realize that diagnosis according to TCHM differs greatly from Western diagnosis. To understand this, consider two hypothetical patients with the single Western diagnosis of migraine headaches. The first might be said to have "dryness in the liver and ascending Qi," while another might be diagnosed with "exogenous wind-cold." Based on these differing diagnoses, entirely different remedies might be applied. In other words, there is no such thing as a TCHM remedy for migraines per se; rather, treatment must be individualized to the imbalance determined by traditional theory.

The herbal formulas used in TCHM consist of four categories of herbs: ministerial, deputy, assistant, and envoy. The ministerial herb addresses the principal pattern of the disease. Deputy herbs assist the ministerial herb or address coexisting conditions. Assistant herbs are designed to reduce the side effects of the first two classes of herbs, and envoy herbs direct the therapy to a particular part of the body. For example, in the case of "dryness in the liver and ascending Qi" described above, an herbalist might employ a ministerial herb to reverse ascending Qi, a deputy herb to exert a moistening effect, an assistant herb to prevent the stagnation of Qi (Qi stagnation is said to be a side effect of moistening herbs), and an envoy to carry these effects to the liver.

TCHM remedies can also be designed to fit all common causes of migraines simultaneously, mostly by multiplying the number of ingredients. Practitioners of TCHM frown upon this "one-size-fits-all" approach, but it is often popular among consumers and easier to test scientifically.

Types of Chinese Herbal Remedies
To use Chinese herbal medicine in the most traditional fashion, you must visit an herbalist's shop. There,

experienced herb preparers will chop, grind, fry, and slice dried herbs according to the prescription given by an experienced herbalist. You will walk home with a packet of dried herbs that need to be prepared according to the instructions, which typically involve adding water, boiling for several hours in a ceramic pot, pouring off the liquid, adding more water, and repeating the process twice more. Certain herbs are supposed to be added right at the end, while others require extra-long preparation.

If you don't wish to carry out such a complex process, or if a classic herbal shop is not available, you may wish to move one step away from tradition and purchase an already-prepared Kampo formula. There are several hundred such formulas designed to match the most commonly seen forms of imbalance. Available in powder, capsule, or tablet form, they can be used much more conveniently than fully traditional herbs. Many Kampo combinations are licensed in Japan and are manufactured there on a large scale by reputable manufacturers.

The lowest level of TCHM, scarcely deserving the name at all, involves so-called Chinese Patent Remedies, which consist most commonly of tiny brown spheres in small brown bottles. They are marketed both for classical imbalances and western disease categories. Patent remedies are inexpensive and widely available. However, there have been so many scandals involving dangerous contaminants not listed on the label that we recommend avoiding this form of treatment entirely.

In the West, herbal medicine is part of folk medicine. However, in China there is a distinct tradition of Chinese folk medicine that is separate from the orthodox, rather academic TCHM approach. In this Chinese folk medicine, herbs are used more simply, somewhat in the manner of Western herbal medicine. Herbs most commonly used in this manner include astragalus , dong quai , ginger , kudzu (Pueraria lobata), licorice , lycium , Panax ginseng , and schizandra . For more information on the use of these herbs, see the appropriate individual articles.

Besides herbs, substances that we might consider supplements are utilized in TCHM. These include extract of human placenta, 76 glandular extracts, and a variety of minerals.

What Is Chinese Herbal Medicine Used for Today
In the traditional system of Chinese herbal medicine, herbal formulas can be used to treat virtually any condition. Some of the most common uses in China include liver disease (hepatitis and cirrhosis), sexual dysfunction in men , infertility in women , insomnia , colds and flus , menstrual pain , irregular menstruation, menopause , and cancer treatment support .

Acupuncture is often used along with herbs as a supplemental treatment; in addition, extraordinarily detailed lifestyle suggestions are common. It is not unusual for a traditional practitioner to "prescribe" dinner, as well as counsel changes in living situation (for example, move from the basement to the first floor or face the bed south rather than north). Exercise systems such as Tai Chi and Qigong may also be recommended.

What Is the Scientific Evidence for Traditional Chinese Herbal Medicine

To establish the effectiveness of a treatment, it must be put through a double-blind, placebo-controlled trial . For this reason, our database is organized around such studies. However, there are a few issues that make it a bit difficult to study TCHM in this way.

The first problem involves diagnosis. As described above, there is no such thing as a TCHM remedy for migraine headaches, for example. Each person with migraines receives individualized treatment. This introduces an extra wrinkle for experimenters.

The best way to address this issue is as follows. People are chosen to participate in a study based on a Western diagnosis. Next, all participants are diagnosed by a classic herbal practitioner and prescribed a formula specific to their individual constitutions according to the principles of TCHM. Finally, another party steps in and provides participants with either the real formula or a placebo formula, under conditions whereby neither practitioners nor participants know which is which.

Other studies utilize a fixed remedy for all participants, in hopes that it will still prove effective on average. Such an approach doesn't really test the effectiveness of true TCHM; rather, it tests a much-simplified form of it. Still, trials of this type are valid as far as they go.

Numerous other studies simply involve enrolling people with a certain condition and giving each participant an herbal remedy. Researchers then record the extent of improvement. Such "open label" trials , however, prove virtually nothing because even phony treatments will appear to cause benefits.

Finally, many of these studies were performed in China, and, up to the time of this writing, research on Chinese medicine conducted in China generally falls far short of modern scientific standards of rigor.

Chronic Hepatitis

Hepatitis is a serious problem in many Asian countries, and conventional care leaves much to be desired. For this reason, herbal remedies are widely used.

The herbal combination Shosaiko-to (Minor Bupleurum) has been approved as a treatment for chronic hepatitis by the Japanese Health Ministry, and it enjoys wide use in that country and elsewhere. However, a search of the literature uncovered only one large-scale, double-blind, placebo-controlled study supporting its effectiveness. In this 24-week trial, the efficacy of Shosaiko-to was tested in 222 people with chronic active hepatitis using a double-blind, placebo-controlled crossover design. Results showed that use of Shosaiko-to significantly improved liver function measurements compared to placebo. Although these results are promising, an absence of long-term evaluation limits their meaningfulness.

Other Chinese herbal remedies have been tested as adjuncts to conventional interferon treatment with promising results. However, published trials are of generally poor quality.

Note: If you are on interferon therapy, you should not use Chinese herbal formulas (or any herbs or supplements) except under the supervision of a physician.

Combination Chinese herbal therapies have also shown a bit of promise for the treatment of chronic hepatitis; tested formulas include Bing Gan Tang, Yi Zhu decoction, Fuzheng Jiedu Tang, and Jianpi Wenshen recipe. However, the quality of most of these studies was again quite poor—the results are mixed and overall, the evidence for these remedies remains far too weak to rely upon. Two studies failed to find Chinese herbal treatment helpful for hepatitis C.

Note: There have been numerous cases of hepatitis and other forms of liver injury caused by Chinese herbs.

Liver Cirrhosis
Shosaiko-to, mentioned in the previous section, has also shown some promise for preventing liver cancer and

liver fibrosis in people with liver cirrhosis or chronic hepatitis. However, the evidence remains marginal. For example, in a double-blind, placebo-controlled study, 260 people with cirrhosis were randomly assigned to take Shosaiko-to or placebo, along with conventional treatment. Over 5 years of evaluation, people taking the herb appeared to be less likely to develop cancer or die, but the results just missed the ordinary cutoff for statistical significance . For the subgroup of participants without hepatitis B infection, the benefits were statistically significant at the usual cutoff point.

Irritable Bowel Syndrome
In a double-blind, placebo-controlled trial, 116 people with irritable bowel syndrome (IBS) were randomly assigned to receive individualized Chinese herbal formulations, a "one-size-fits-all" Chinese herbal formulation, or placebo. Treatment consisted of 5 capsules 3 times daily, taken for 16 weeks. The results showed that both forms of active treatment were superior to placebo, significantly reducing IBS symptoms. However, the individualized treatment was no more

effective than the "generic" treatment. Similar results were seen in another study as well.

Constipation

The Kampo formula known as Daio-kanzo-to is a mixture of rhubarb and licorice. In a 2-week, double-blind, placebo-controlled trial, 132 people complaining of constipation were randomly assigned to one of three groups: placebo, low-dose Daio-kanzo-to, or high-dose Daio-kanzo-to. The results indicate that the higher-dose group, but not the lower-dose group, experienced statistically significant improvements in constipation compared to placebo.

Allergies

In a double-blind, placebo-controlled trial, 220 people with allergic rhinitis were given either placebo or the Kampo remedy Sho-seiryu-to for a period of 2 weeks. The results showed that use of the herbal formula significantly relieved all major symptoms of allergic rhinitis compared to placebo. Based on this and other more preliminary studies, Sho-seiryu-to has been approved by the Japanese Health Ministry for the treatment of allergic rhinitis and allergic conjunctivitis.

Another combination herbal therapy has shown promise for allergic rhinitis as well. In a 12-week, double-blind, placebo-controlled trial, 58 people with allergic rhinitis were given either placebo or an 11-herb combination remedy called Biminne. This combination therapy contains the following herbs.

- Rehmannia glutinosa
- Scutellaria baicalensis
- Polygonatum sibiricum
- Ginkgo biloba
- Epimedium sagittatum
- Psoralea corylifolia
- Schisandra chinensis
- Prunus mume
- Ledebouriella divaricata
- Angelica dahurica
- Astragalus membranaceus

Use of Biminne produced significant improvements in some symptoms of allergic rhinitis, while other symptoms showed a trend toward improvement that was not statistically significant. A follow-up evaluation suggested that the results persisted for a year after treatment was stopped.

Benefits have been seen in small studies of other formulations as well. However, one study failed to find that use of herbal treatments augmented the effectiveness of acupuncture for allergic rhinitis.

Osteoarthritis

A double-blind, placebo-controlled study of 96 people with osteoarthritis of the knee tested the effectiveness of a mixture of three Chinese herbs (Clematis mandshurica , Trichosanthes kirilowii , and Prunella vulgaris). Participants were randomly assigned to placebo group or one of three other groups: 200 mg, 400 mg, or 600 mg of the herbal formula 3 times daily. After 4 weeks of treatment, significant improvement in arthritis symptoms was seen in all three treatment groups compared to placebo. No dose appeared conclusively superior to the others.

Muscle Spasms

The Kampo remedy Shakuyaku-kanzo-to is a combination of peony root and licorice , commonly used for the treatment of muscle spasms in general. In a double-blind, placebo-controlled study, 101 people with liver cirrhosis who also suffered from severe muscular spasms at least twice per week were given either Shakuyaku-kanzo-to or placebo 3 times daily for 2 weeks. (The herb combination is not specifically aimed at liver cirrhosis. However, people with liver cirrhosis often have muscle spasms, so it made sense to try an anti-muscle-spasm formula on them.) The results showed significant reduction in frequency and severity of spasms among the participants using the herb compared to those taking placebo. However, some participants using the herb developed edema (swelling caused by excess fluid) and weight gain. Researchers attributed this side effect to the licorice constituent.

Menstrual Pain

In a double-blind trial of 40 women complaining of menstrual pain , the Kampo formula Toki-shakuyaku-san was compared to placebo with good results. The design of this study was interesting because researchers preselected women who, according to the principles of traditional Chinese medicine, would be expected to respond to this Kampo treatment. Over six menstrual cycles, women using the real herbal formula experienced significantly less menstrual pain compared to those in the placebo group. Benefits took three menstrual cycles to develop.

In a 2008 review of 39 randomized controlled trials involving a total of 3,475 women, researchers concluded that the use of traditional Chinese herbs shows some promise in for the treatment of menstrual pain. However, firm conclusions were not possible due to the wide variability of study design and herbs used, as well as the poor quality of many of the studies.

Diabetes

A double-blind study of more than 200 people evaluated the effectiveness of Coptis Formula (a traditional combination therapy) with or without the drug glibenclamide for the treatment of diabetes . Coptis Formula appeared to significantly enhance the effectiveness of the drug; however, the herbs produced marginal benefits at best when taken alone.

Asthma

The Kampo remedy Saiboku-to has been approved by the Japanese Health Ministry for the treatment of asthma . However, meaningful supporting evidence appears to be limited to one small trial. In this double-blind, placebo-controlled crossover study, 33 people with mild to moderate asthma received Saiboku-to or placebo 3 times daily for 4 weeks. Treatment with the herbal remedy improved symptoms of asthma to a greater extent than placebo. Additional measurements suggested that Saiboku-to works by reducing asthmatic inflammation (technically, eosinophilia)

A Chinese study using a proprietary formulation reported benefits as well.

Eczema

A Chinese herbal mixture sold under the name Zemaphyte has shown promise as a treatment for eczema . This formula, based on herbs traditionally used for skin conditions, contains the following:

- Ledebouriella seseloides
- Potentilla chinensis
- Akebia clematidis
- Rehmannia glutinosa
- Paeonia lactiflora
- Lophatherum gracile
- Dictamnus dasycarpus
- Tribulus terrestris
- Glycyrrhiza uralensis
- Schizonepeta tenuifolia

In paired double-blind, placebo-controlled trials carried out by one research group, Zemaphyte produced significantly better effects than placebo for both adults and children. Each study enrolled approximately 40 people and used a crossover design in which all participants received the real treatment and placebo for 8 weeks each. Use of the herb significantly reduced eczema symptoms compared to placebo.

However, a subsequent study of similar design performed by a different research group failed to find significant benefit with Zemaphyte. The reason for this discrepancy is not clear.

In a 12-week, double-blind study, a different traditional Chinese herbal formula also failed to prove more effective than placebo for treatment of eczema.

Tension Headache
A topical ointment known as Tiger Balm is a popular treatment for headaches and other conditions. Tiger Balm contains camphor, menthol, cajaput, and clove oil. A double-blind study enrolling 57 people with acute tension headache compared the application of Tiger Balm to the forehead against placebo ointment, as well as against the drug acetaminophen (Tylenol). The

placebo ointment contained mint essence to make it smell similar to Tiger Balm. Real Tiger Balm proved more effective than placebo, and just as effective and more rapid-acting than acetaminophen.

HIV

Chinese herbal therapies have been investigated for the treatment of HIV , but the results have not been very promising. In a 12-week, double-blind, placebo-controlled trial, 30 HIV-infected adults with CD4 counts of 200 to 500 were given a Chinese herbal formula containing 31 herbs. The results hint that use of the herbal combination might have improved various symptoms compared to placebo, but none of the differences were statistically significant. Interestingly, people who believed they were taking the real treatment showed significant benefit regardless of whether they were in the placebo group or the real treatment group.

In another double-blind, placebo-controlled trial, 68 HIV-infected adults were given either placebo or a preparation of 35 Chinese herbs for a period of 6 months. The results indicate that use of Chinese herbs did not improve symptoms or objective measurements of HIV severity. In fact, people using the herbs reported more digestive problems than those given placebo!

Cancer Treatment

Chemotherapy

A double-blind study performed in Hong Kong evaluated the potential benefits in cancer chemotherapy of personalized herbal formulas designed according to the principles of Traditional Chinese herbal medicine. In this study, 120 people undergoing chemotherapy for early-stage breast or colon cancer were given either a personalized formula or placebo. Researchers evaluated numerous possible effects of the treatment, but found benefits in only one: reduction of nausea. Note that even this single result is less meaningful than it may seem; it is statistical questionable to use a multiplicity of outcome measures. A review of 15 mostly poor quality trials with 862 patients suggested that Chinese herbal medicine might improve quality of life in patients with non-small cell lung cancer undergoing chemotherapy.

Prostate Cancer

For several years, the Chinese herbal combination PC-SPES underwent significant investigation as a treatment for prostate cancer, with apparently impressive results. However, subsequent investigation revealed that PC-SPES contained undisclosed pharmaceutical ingredients (principally, a form of estrogen and the strong blood thinner Coumadin), and that these were probably responsible for its benefits. The treatment has since been withdrawn.

Liver Cancer

Numerous studies have evaluated traditional Chinese herbal medicine for treatment of liver cancer with generally positive results. However, study design and reporting were markedly substandard.

Breast Cancer

After a mastectomy, some women develop wound complications. Ninety women who had undergone a mastectomy were randomized to receive 1 of 3 treatments: routine wound care, the Chinese herb Salvia miltiorrhiza (given intravenously for 3 days), or another Chinese herb called anisodamine (also given intravenously for 3 days). The women who received the herbal treatments had fewer wound complications compared to those in the routine wound care group. But, the women who took anisodamine had more adverse effects related to the treatment, like painful urination.

Other Uses for Traditional Chinese Herbal Medicine

A large, double-blind study conducted in China reported that use of the traditional remedy xue-zhi-kang by people with a previous history of a heart attack could reduce the risk that they would suffer a subsequent severe cardiovascular problem, such as a stroke or another heart attack. Chinese herbal medicine may also be helpful for people with angina. In a small, randomized trial of 66 adults with stable angina, Shenshao tablets (containing ginsenosides and white peony) reduced the frequency of angina attacks.

In a small, double-blind, placebo-controlled trial, use of the herbal combination Banxia Houpo Tang (also called Hange Koboku-To or Magnolia and Pinelliae Formula) was tested for the treatment of impaired cough reflex in people who had suffered a stroke . The results indicated that the herbal combination was more effective than placebo treatment for improving the coughing response. In another study, 140 people who recently had a stroke were randomized to receive the herbal formula sanchitongshu (200 mg three times daily) plus aspirin (50 mg once daily) or aspirin plus placebo. 88 After one month of treatment, those in the herbal formula group had a greater improvement in their neurological deficits and activities of daily living compared to the aspirin plus placebo group.

While traditional Chinese herbal medicine has a long history of use for infertility, there is not a lot of strong evidence to support its effectiveness. In a 2011 review of 14 randomized trials involving 1,316 women, the addition of Chinese herbal medicine to the prescription medication clomiphene (used to induce ovulation) was associated with increased pregnancy rates. 89 The researchers pointed out, though, that the studies were of poor quality with low sample sizes. As with the earlier review, a 2012 analysis of 30 studies, including 8 randomized trials, also found evidence to support the use of Chinese herbal medicine for improving pregnancy rates.91 This review included trials that compared Chinese herbal medicine alone, with acupuncture, or with standard drug therapy to drug therapy alone. While the researchers concluded that Chinese herbal medicine may improve pregnancy rates , as with the previous review, the quality of the studies was questionable.

Various Chinese herbal formulas have been evaluated for the treatment of respiratory infections. The results of published studies appear to indicate that these formulas are more effective than standard antibiotics, but the poor design of most of these trials precludes placing much faith in their outcomes. One combination therapy called Shuang Huang Lian has better supporting evidence than most.

A review of 17 trials found that there is limited evidence to support the use of Traditional Chinese herbal preparations for the common cold . Although reliable evidence supporting the benefits of Traditional Chinese herbs alone for the treatment of influenza is lacking, a randomized trial involving 410 people with H1N1 influenza found that those who took a combination of 12 Chinese herbal medicines (maxingshigan-yinqiaosan, 200 mL, 4 times daily) along with the antiviral medication oseltamivir (75 mg twice daily) for five days experienced a more rapid resolution of fever compared to those taking oseltamivir alone. One double-blind, placebo-controlled study tested the remedy Hochu-ekki-to for enhancing immune response to influenza vaccine, but failed to find benefit.

One study evaluated the effectiveness of an herbal combination containing herbs commonly used for the treatment of cough , but failed to find the treatment effective. (Note: This study has been incorrectly reported as finding the tested treatment effective; indeed, use of the treatment did help suppress coughing, but so did the placebo treatment, and there was no significant differences between the groups.)

A double-blind, placebo-controlled study of 29 people with chronic fatigue syndrome found indications that use of the Kampo remedy Hochu-ekki-to significantly improved symptoms compared to placebo.

In one study, the herbal formula Duhuo Jisheng Wan, widely used for osteoarthritis , proved to be as effective as the standard anti-inflammatory drug diclofenac. However, the herb caused as many side effects as the drug, and was slower to act. (It was so slow, in fact, that its benefits could have been due solely to the placebo effect.) This study did not use a placebo control group.

The Kampo remedies Saiko-keishi-to and Shosaiko-to have been suggested for the treatment of epilepsy , but the supporting evidence is too preliminary to be relied upon. Both of these combination treatments consist of bupleurum, peony root, pinellia root, cassia bark, ginger root , jujube fruit, Asian ginseng root , Asian scullcap root, and licorice root , but the proportions are different.

In a review of 21 studies involving almost 3,000 subjects, researchers concluded that Chinese herbs were as effective as commonly prescribed medications for drug withdrawal symptoms in heroin addicts . They could not draw any conclusions, however, regarding which specific herbs were more most beneficial.

One study quoted as showing that a Chinese herbal formula can reduce blood pressure actually failed to find any effect on blood pressure.

Tripterygium hypoglaucum hutch, another type of herb that is used in TCHM, was found in one study to provide added benefit in treating hives when given along with the medication cetirizine.

Other traditional herbal combinations with some supporting evidence (often from studies of questionable quality) include Xiao-Yao-San (Free and Easy Wanderer) for depression and bipolar syndrome , Mai-Men-Dong-Tang for allergic asthma , Yi-Gan San for dementia , Bofu-tsusho-san for weight loss and diabetes , Chang Ji Tai for irritable bowel syndrome , and Ondamtanggamibang (a Korean formulation) for reducing symptoms of stress . Qinzhu Liangxue for psoriasis , and red peony root for acute pancreatitis .

How to Choose a Practitioner of Traditional Chinese Herbal Medicine

There is no general certification for the practice of TCHM. Many people who are certified in acupuncture , however, have significant training in herbal medicine as well. (In general, 500 hours of specific training is considered necessary.) Some states offer the license of OMD (Doctor of Oriental Medicine); licensed OMDs are generally well versed in TCHM.

Safety Issues

There are several serious safety concerns with the use of TCHM.

One concern involves the use of multiple herbs typical in this approach. In general, conventional medicine makes a point of using as few medications as possible (in theory, at least) because the greater the number of medications, the greater the risk of harm. (Also, when medications are used together and harm does result, it's hard to know which drug was at fault.) From this perspective, formulas consisting of 5, 10, or 30 herbs are quite worrisome.

Interestingly, such combinations are actually designed for the purpose of reducing risks. According to TCHM theory, the various herbs in a formula balance and moderate each other. Unfortunately, this theory has never been put to the test, and there are reasons not to trust it. Simply put, it is very difficult to get an accurate picture of the risks of a treatment if you don't keep systematic records of adverse effects, and the ancient Chinese government had no such system in place. In any case, the individualized nature of treatment would make it almost impossible to track harm. Herbalists would be expected to notice immediate, dramatic reactions to herbal formulas, and one can assume with some confidence that treatments used for thousands of years are at least unlikely to cause such problems in very many people who take them. However, certain types of harm could be expected to easily elude the detection of traditional herbalists. These include safety problems that are delayed, occur relatively rarely, or are difficult to detect without scientific instruments. How would a traditional herbalist ever know, for example, if a treatment caused liver failure in one out of 100,000 people who used it, especially if such failure took 2 or more years to develop? If such a death did occur in the herbalist's patient population, it would probably be attributed to hepatitis or some other common cause.

These factors may explain why Chinese herbal medicine traditionally uses treatments that are now recognized as potentially dangerous, such as mercury, arsenic, lead, licorice, coltsfoot, and Aristolochia.

Mercury, arsenic, and lead accumulate slowly in the body, and for many years their harm can only be detected by lab tests. Licorice (used in many herb formulas to "harmonize" the ingredients) can raise blood pressure and disturb blood chemistry. These effects were presumably undetectable to traditional practitioners unless they became quite severe. The herb Aristolochia can cause severe kidney damage and kidney cancer, but only rarely. Modern medical surveillance has uncovered quite a few such cases, but traditional herbology considered the herb worth using. Aristolochia contains aristolochic acid, a substance shown in animal studies to damage the kidney when taken in high enough doses.

Chinese herbal products generally list Aristolochia on the label when it is present, but in some cases, Aristolochia was apparently added accidentally it is similar in appearance to a much safer herb.

Coltsfoot (Tussilago farfara), used in Chinese cough syrups and other formulations, contains pyrrolizidine alkaloids, substances that can over time damage the liver. This also does not appear to have been noticed by traditional herbalists. Under modern conditions of medical surveillance, many incidents have been reported in which use of Chinese herbs appears to have various forms of liver injury, including acute hepatitis, chronic hepatitis, hepatic fibrosis, and acute liver failure. Ancient herbal practitioners might not have been able to distinguish these herb-induced illnesses from the effects of infectious hepatitis, a widely prevalent condition, and thereby failed to make the connection; even today, in fact, it appears that many cases of liver failure attributed to hepatitis have in fact been caused by the Chinese herbs used to treat hepatitis!

Other reported complications of Chinese herbal treatments include movement disorders and ovarian failure.

Another set of potential problems arises from the fact that Chinese herbal medicine does not restrict itself to plant products with subtle effects. Many traditional Chinese herbal remedies are, simply put, poisons. When taken in proper doses, they may be safe for use, but dosage miscalculation or use in a particularly susceptible person may lead to serious consequences, including death. For example, in Hong Kong, poisoning caused by the herb aconite (used in numerous Chinese herbal formulas) was sufficiently widespread that public health authorities felt it necessary to launch an information campaign to combat the problem.

Besides toxicity caused by Chinese herbs, other problems have been caused by adulteration of herbal products with unlisted ingredients. 36 For example, the Chinese herbal formula PC-SPES, used for prostate cancer, turned out to contain three pharmaceutical drug diethylstilbestrol (DES), warfarin (Coumadin), and indomethacin. This appears to have been an intentional adulteration designed somewhat along the lines of a traditional Chinese formula, with one pharmaceutical adulterant that treated prostate cancer balanced by two others to offset the side effects of the first. Unfortunately, the combination is dangerous and has caused at least one case of severe bleeding.

In another episode, 8 out of 11 Chinese herbal creams sold in the United Kingdom for the treatment of eczema were found to contain strong pharmaceutical steroids. Other studies have also found steroids in eczema preparations. In addition, Chinese herbal weight loss aids have also been found to contain an unlisted chemical related to the appetite suppressant drug fenfluramine (of fen-phen fame).

Herbal products approved by the Japanese government have undergone meaningful safety testing and are very unlikely to contain known toxins or unlisted drugs. However, this does not mean they are completely safe. For example, several case reports suggest that therapy for chronic hepatitis combining an approved herbal formula with the standard drug interferon can cause severe inflammation of the lungs.

The herbal formulas Takeda Kampo Ichoyaku K-matsu, Taisho Kampo Ichoyaku, and Kanebo Kampo Ichoyaku Hused, all used to treat upset stomach, might reduce the effectiveness of the Parkinson's disease medication levodopa.

Commonly-Used Chinese Herbs

Astragalus (huangqi)

The long tap roots of astragalus are, today, the most commonly used herb material in China. Astragalus normalizes immune responses (used for immune deficiency, allergies, and autoimmunity), benefits digestive functions, and treats disorders of the skin from burns to carbuncles. Astragalus is used as a promoter of the functions of several other herbs, such as salvia and tang-kuei . It is used in the treatment of AIDS and hepatitis, for chronic colitis, senility, and cardiovascular diseases. Cancer patients who take this herb can often avoid the white blood cell deficiencies (leukopenia) that occur with chemotherapy. The root is rich in polysaccharides and flavonoids that produce the beneficial effects. Astragalus may be used by itself, usually as a liquid extract, or in combination with other herbs in the form of teas, pills, or tablets. Dosage is from 1-60 grams per day, depending on the application and form. Caution: some individuals may experience flatulence and abdominal bloating from use of astragalus.

Atractylodes (baizhu)
The rhizomes of atractylodes are considered very important to the treatment of digestive disorders and problems of moisture accumulation. The herb helps move moisture (and nutrients) from the digestive tract to the blood, reducing problems of diarrhea, gas, and bloating, and helps move moisture from the body tissues to the bladder for elimination, alleviating edema. The herb is frequently included in tonic prescriptions, and the herb is rarely used by itself. Dosage is from 200 milligrams in capsules and tablets to 15 grams per day in the form of decoction. Caution: persons suffering from a

hot and dry condition may experience worsening of those symptoms if large amounts of atractylodes are used.

Bupleurum (chaihu)

The thin roots of bupleurum are one of the most frequently used herbs in the Japanese practice of Oriental medicine. Doctors in Japan have found it useful in the treatment of liver diseases, skin ailments, arthritis, menopausal syndrome, withdrawal from corticosteroid use, nephritis, stress-induced ulcers, and mental disorders. The roots are rich in saponins that reduce inflammation and regulate hormone levels. The herb is not used by itself, but rather in formulas with about four to twelve ingredients, made as teas, pills, or tablets. Dosage ranges from a few hundred milligrams of powder to about 15 grams in tea per day. Caution: some individuals may experience dizziness or headaches from use of bupleurum.

Cinnamon (guizhi and rougi)

The twigs (guizhi) and bark (rougi) of this large tropical tree are said to warm the body, invigorate the circulation, and harmonize the energy of the upper and lower body.

Modern studies demonstrate that cinnamon reduces allergy reactions. Traditionally, cinnamon twig is used when the peripheral circulation is poor and cinnamon bark is used when the entire body is cold. If the upper body is warm and the lower body is cold, then cinnamon will correct the imbalance. Cinnamon is usually cooked together with other herbs to make a warming tea, or powdered with other herbs to make a pill or tablet that regulates circulation of blood. Dosage is 0.3-3 grams of bark and up to 9 grams of twig per day. Caution: large amounts of cinnamon are irritating to the liver and should not be used by those with inflammatory liver disorders.

Coptis (huanglian)
This rhizome (underground stem) is one of the most bitter herbs used in Chinese medicine. It is rich in alkaloids that inhibit infections and calm nervous agitation; it is usually combined with other bitter-tasting herbs, such as phellodendron, scute, and gardenia, to promote these actions. Examples of its many uses include treatment of skin diseases, intestinal infections,

hypertension, and insomnia. Coptis is a close relative of an extremely bitter and very useful American herb, goldenseal. Because of its taste, coptis is most often used in the form of pills or tablets. Typical dosage is from a few hundred milligrams of powder to 3 grams in decoction per day. Caution: regular use of coptis in large dosage may cause diarrhea.

Ginger (jiang)

The fibrous rhizome of this herb is highly spicy and said to benefit digestion, neutralize poisons in food, ventilate the lungs, and warm the circulation to the limbs. Today, ginger is commonly used as a spice in cooking; as a medicine it has been shown helpful in counteracting nausea from various causes including morning sickness, motion sickness, and food contamination. Many herbalists use ginger in the treatment of cough (it acts as an expectorant) and common cold. Ginger is used in making teas and the powder is encapsulated for easy consumption. Typical dosage is from a few milligrams used as an assistant in herb formulas to about 3 grams per day in making decoctions. Instant tea granules (sugar or honey base) are available. Caution: persons who suffer from dryness-dry cough, thirst, dry constipation, etc.- may find that ginger worsens the condition.

Ginseng (renshen)
The root has long been cherished as a disease-preventive and a life preserver. It calms the spirit, nourishes the viscera, and helps one gain wisdom. Modern applications include normalizing blood pressure, regulating blood sugar, resisting fatigue, increasing oxygen utilization, and enhancing immune functions. Traditionally, the root is cooked in a double boiler to make a tea, used either alone or with several other herbs. Today, teas can be made quickly from carefully prepared extracts in liquid or dry form; ginseng powder is made into tablets or encapsulated, and ginseng formulas are available in numerous forms for easy consumption. Typical dosage is 0.5-3.0 grams. Higher doses may be used over the short term for specific therapeutic actions: in China 30 grams is recommended to treat shock (sudden hypotension). Caution: excessive consumption of ginseng can lead to

nervousness and may produce hormonal imbalance in women.

Hoelen (fuling)

This herb is a large fungus that grows on pine roots. It is used to alleviate irritation of the gastro-intestinal system and, like atractylodes, it helps transport moisture out of the digestive system into the blood stream and from the various body tissues to the bladder. When bits of the pine root are included in the herb material it is called fushen; the combination of the fungus and pine produces a mild sedative action. This herb, because it is quite mild, is mostly used in making decoctions or dried decoctions, with a dosage equivalent of about 10-15 grams per day. The herb is non-toxic and rarely causes any adverse effects.

Licorice (gancao)

The roots have an extremely sweet taste (but are also bitter) and are said to neutralize toxins, relieve inflammation, and enhance digestion. In Europe, a drug has been made from licorice extract that heals gastric ulcers. Licorice is used by Chinese doctors in the treatment of hepatitis, sore throat, muscle spasms, and, when baked with honey, for treatment hyperthyroidism and heart valve diseases. Traditionally, licorice is thought to enhance the effectiveness of herb formulas and is used to moderate the flavor of herb teas; as a result, it is found in about one-third of all Chinese herb prescriptions. Licorice powder is encapsulated for easy consumption or mixed with other herbs and tableted. Dosage is from very small amounts (a few hundred milligrams) to 15 grams per day in decoction used to treat viral hepatitis. Caution: excessive consumption of licorice over an extended period to time can cause sodium/potassium imbalance with symptoms of tachycardia and/or edema.

Ma-huang (mahuang)
The stem-like leaves when taken in a dose of several grams stimulate perspiration, open the breathing passages, and invigorate the central nervous system energy. It has been shown that most of these effects are due to two alkaloid components, ephedrine and pseudoephedrine, both of them having been made into

modern drugs (for asthma and sinus congestion, respectively). In addition, the stimulating action of ma-huang has led to its use as a metabolic enhancer (burns calories more quickly) for those who are trying to lose weight. Ma-huang also has anti-inflammatory actions useful in treating some cases of arthralgia and myalgia. Ma-huang can be made into a tea, or used in extract form; powdered ma-huang is rarely used. Dosage range is 1-9 grams/day, usually in two or three divided doses. Caution: the stimulant effect of ma-huang can cause insomnia and agitation; persons with very high blood pressure may find this symptom worsened by use of ma-huang.

Peony (baishao and chihshao)
The root of this common flower is used to regulate the blood. It relaxes the blood vessels, reduces platelet sticking, nourishes the blood, and promotes circulation to the skin and extremities. The root of both wild and cultivated peonies are used. The wild peony yields "red peony" (chihshao) a fibrous root that is especially used

for stimulating blood circulation. The cultivated peony yields "white peony" (baishao) a dense root that nourishes the blood. Peony is often combined with tang-kuei, licorice, or other herbs mentioned here to enhance or control their effects. The dosage range is from 0.5-15 grams per day. Peony rarely causes any adverse reactions.

Rehmannia (dihuang)
The root of this herb is a dark, moist herb that is extensively used to nourish the blood and the hormonal system. It is frequently used in the treatment of problems of aging, because of its ability to restore the levels of several declining hormones. There are two forms of the herb that are currently used: one, designated shengdihuang or raw rehmannia, is given to reduce inflammation and is included in many formulas for autoimmune disorders; the other is designated shoudihuang or cooked rehmannia, and is used as a nourishing tonic. Often, the two forms are combined together in equal proportions to address inflammatory problems that are related to the lack of adequate levels of

regulating hormones. The herb is mainly used in making decoctions or dried decoctions, with a dosage of 10-30 grams per day. Caution: persons with weak digestion and tendency to experience loose stool or diarrhea may find that this herb, especially cooked rehmannia, worsens those symptoms.

Rhubarb (dahuang)

This large root was one of the first herbs that the Western world imported from China. It serves as a very reliable laxative, and also has other benefits: enhancing appetite when taken before meals in small amounts, promoting blood circulation and relieving pain in cases of injury or inflammation, and inhibiting intestinal infections. Rhubarb also reduces autoimmune reactions. The impact of rhubarb is influenced by how it is prepared; if it is cooked for a long period of time, the laxative actions are reduced but other actions are retained. Typical dosage is 0.5-3 grams per day. Caution: rhubarb, alone or in formulas, should not be used by those with irritable bowel conditions, as it may cause cramping and diarrhea.

Salvia (danshen)

The deep red roots of this Chinese sage plant have become an important herb during the past two decades even though it was used for centuries before that. It is applied in almost all cases where the body tissues have been damaged by disease or injury; thus, it is given for post-stroke syndrome, traumatic injury, chronic inflammation and/or infection, and degenerative diseases. It is best known for its ability to promote circulation in the capillary beds-the so-called microcirculation system. In addition, salvia lowers blood pressure, helps reduce cholesterol, and enhances function of the liver. It may be consumed alone or with other herbs, in wines, teas, pills, or tablets; dosage is 1-20 grams per day. Salvia rarely causes any adverse reactions.

Tang-kuei (danggui)

The root has been long respected as a blood-nourishing agent. It has its highest rate of use among women because tang-kuei will help to regulate uterine blood flow and contraction, but when employed in complex formulas it can be used by both men and women to nourish the blood, moisten the intestines, improve the circulation, calm tension, and relieve pain. Tang-kuei is frequently said to have estrogenic effects, but this is not a valid claim. The recommended dosage for tang-kuei is 0.5-9 grams per day. Tang-kuei may be made as a tea or cooked with chicken to make soup (the taste is quite strong), but it is often used today as a powder, encapsulated or made into tablets, alone or with other herbs. Caution: some individuals find that tang-kuei causes nausea or loose stool.

Examples Of Herb Combining To Make An Effective Treatment

An ancient formula prescribed for the initial stage of an infectious disease is Cinnamon Combination. It includes cinnamon, peony, licorice, and ginger. It is said that the cinnamon (twig) and peony coordinate the circulation at the surface of the body (where disease is believed to enter) and relaxes tense muscles. Ginger and licorice improve the digestive functions and improve the body's healing energy. An ancient formula used to treat chronic illness is Ginseng and Tang-kuei Ten Combination. It includes astragalus, ginseng, atractylodes, hoelen, licorice, cinnamon, tang-kuei, peony, and rehmannia. Astragalus, ginseng, atractylodes, hoelen, and licorice promote digestive functions, increase the energy, nourish the internal organs, and enhance weakened immune responses. Cinnamon (bark) warms up the weakened metabolism. Tang-kuei, peony, and rehmannia nourish the blood. Another ancient formula, used for a variety of diseases and function disorders, is Minor Bupleurum Combination. It includes bupleurum, ginseng, ginger, hoelen, and licorice. Bupleurum harmonizes the circulation between the internal organs and the body surface, it alleviates stress in the chest and abdomen, and it reduces inflammation. As indicated above, ginseng, ginger, hoelen, and licorice benefit the digestive processes and increase energy.

All of these formulas are widely used today, often by making some slight modifications to address the particular needs of the individual or the characteristics of the disease. For example, Cinnamon Combination (with appropriate modifications) has been used in Chinese clinical trials for treatment of frostbite, pernicious vomiting of pregnancy, and appendicitis. Ginseng and Tang-kuei Ten Combination has been applied to treatment of side-effects of cancer therapy and for prevention of cancer recurrence after successful treatment. Minor Bupleurum Combination is one of the formulas frequently given in cases of chronic hepatitis B infection, and it is also used for inflammation of the stomach and pancreas.

Conclusion

Experts believe it's safe, if you go to someone who knows what he's doing. This is especially true of acupuncture, tai chi, cupping, and moxibustion.

Herbs can be a little trickier. They don't go through the same FDA process as drugs. That means there's not as much research on them, and it can be hard to know exactly what's in them. Plus, herbs can have side effects or impact other medicine you're taking. Again, it's important to go to someone who really understands her practice. And always check with your doctor first.

TCM is an approach that covers a lot of ground, and results vary. The practices haven't been studied in the same way as Western medicine. More research has been done on herbs and acupuncture than other treatments. But studies show a lot of promise:

Acupuncture is commonly accepted as a treatment for a number of conditions, including pain relief and limiting side effects from chemotherapy.

A number of herbs used in TCM are also used at well-respected, Western medicine clinics to treat anything from trouble sleeping to arthritis to menopause.

Tai chi seems to improve balance in people with Parkinson's disease.

Cupping may help relieve pain from shingles.

In general, doctors suggest you don't use it to totally replace Western medicine, especially if you have a serious condition like cancer or liver disease.

They also urge caution, especially with herbs, if you're:

- Elderly
- Pregnant or breastfeeding
- Scheduled for surgery (some herbs could lead to bleeding problems or prevent drugs used during surgery from working)
- Taking other medicine as well
- Treating a child

www.ingramcontent.com/pod-product-compliance
Lightning Source LLC
Chambersburg PA
CBHW070321160726
47999CB00003B/1094